MCQs for MRCOphth

(Membership of the Royal College of Ophthalmologists examinations)

by **Ivor S Levy**
Consultant Ophthalmic Surgeon, The Royal London and Moorfields Eye Hospitals; Consultant Neuro-Ophthalmologist, The Royal London Hospital

and **Paul Riordan-Eva**
Senior Registrar in Neuro-Ophthalmology, The National Hospital, Queen Square, London

D1333934

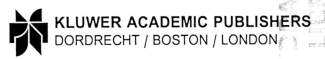

KLUWER ACADEMIC PUBLISHERS
DORDRECHT / BOSTON / LONDON

Distributors

for the United States and Canada: Kluwer Academic Publishers, PO Box 358, Accord Station, Hingham, MA 02018-0358, USA
for all other countries: Kluwer Academic Publishers Group, Distribution Center, PO Box 322, 3300 AH Dordrecht, The Netherlands

ISBN 0-7923-8848-8

A catalogue record for this book is available from the British Library.

Published in the United Kingdom by Kluwer Academic Publishers, PO Box 55, Lancaster, UK.

Kluwer Academic Publishers BV incorporates the publishing programmes of D. Reidel, Martinus Nijhoff, Dr W. Junk and MTP Press.

Printed and bound in Great Britain by Hartnolls Ltd., Bodmin, Cornwall.

Contents

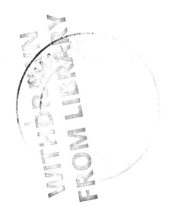

Foreword

One of the most challenging tasks in a junior doctor's specialist training is the final professional examination in the chosen speciality.

The syllabus and specific requirements regarding eligibility to sit the examination have been carefully laid down by the respective Colleges in an attempt to set the required standards of professional skill and ability. The format of the examination itself has been selected in order to thoroughly test these standards.

These examinations are a necessary hurdle to overcome. Thorough preparation is essential; the information gleaned and stored will form the foundation of the candidate's specialist knowledge.

To be aware of the nature of the questions likely to be posed and how best to approach the answers is helpful. This series of publications of Multiple Choice Questions is aimed at candidates preparing for the College of Ophthalmologists Examination. In setting out a broad range of typical multiple choice questions, their aim is to test the level of the candidates knowledge as well as helping to reinforce specific points and refine examination technique.

Clive Migdal
Consultant Ophthalmologist
Western Eye Hospital, London

July 1993

Introduction

It might be questionable whether further multiple choice question (MCQ) books in ophthalmology are justified. I felt so for three reasons. First, those already published have answers which contain a number of errors. Second, and more importantly, many of the questions and some of the answers are ambiguous. Finally, the other books have a number of questions relating to treatment. Since the medical and surgical aspects of ophthalmology change so rapidly that treatments regarded as 'standard' only ten years ago are now completely outmoded, such questions are inappropriate.

Whilst I am sure that the present book is not without errors, an attempt has been made to keep these to a very minimum and for this I am most grateful to Mark Batterbury who has diligently and rigorously scrutinized both our questions and answers, correcting errors and pointing out ambiguities. This book would certainly not have been written without my co-author, Paul Riordan-Eva. By putting possible tentative questions to each other we hope we were able to eliminate those unsuitable. We have also tried to ensure that we covered the syllabus of the Royal College of Ophthalmologists. In spite of all these efforts, there may still be errors and ambiguities and I would welcome readers' comments and corrections.

Finally, I would like to thank Dr Peter Clarke of Kluwer Academic Publishers for his constant and close attention to this book.

Ivor S Levy

ANATOMY AND EMBRYOLOGY

1. **Structures derived from embryonic neural ectoderm include:**

A. lens capsule
B. ciliary muscle
C. retinal pigment epithelium
D. levator palpebrae superioris
E. ciliary epithelium

2. **The following structures are situated in the midbrain:**

A. vertical gaze centre
B. sixth nerve nucleus
C. Edinger–Westphal nucleus
D. superior colliculus
E. lateral geniculate nucleus

3. **The following structures pass through the superior orbital fissure:**

A. ophthalmic artery
B. lacrimal branch of the trigeminal nerve
C. abducens nerve
D. superior ophthalmic vein
E. trochlear nerve

4. Cornea:

A. the corneal epithelium is one cell thick
B. Descemet's membrane is the basement layer of the corneal endothelium
C. the corneal stroma is acellular
D. is supplied by the ophthalmic division of the trigeminal nerve
E. its thickness determines the eye's refractive power

5. Optic nerve:

A. each optic nerve contains about 1 million nerve fibres
B. there is no arachnoid mater in the optic nerve meninges
C. myelination is virtually complete at birth
D. the laminar portion of the optic nerve is supplied by branches of the central retinal artery
E. consists of axons of the retinal ganglion cells

6. The medial wall of the orbit:

A. is partly formed by the maxilla
B. forms the lateral wall of the ethmoid sinuses
C. is normally concave with respect to the globe
D. includes foramina for the anterior and posterior ethmoidal vessels
E. is pierced by the nerve that supplies sensation to the tip of the nose

7. The retina:

A. is thickest at the fovea
B. its outer third is avascular
C. retinal vascularization is completed during the sixth month of gestation
D. is separated from the choroid by Bruch's membrane
E. the Müller cells connect the photoreceptors to the ganglion cells

8. Levator palpebrae superioris:

A. arises from the lesser wing of the sphenoid bone
B. has a common embryological origin with the superior rectus muscle
C. attaches to the superior conjunctival fornix
D. is supplied by the facial nerve
E. passes through the orbicularis oculi to insert into the skin of the upper eyelid

9. The anterior cranial fossa:

A. is separated from the orbit by the orbital plate of the frontal bone
B. contains the temporal lobes of the cerebrum
C. its floor includes the roof of the nasal cavity
D. is related to the frontal sinus
E. forms part of the lateral wall of the orbit

10. The crystalline lens:

A.   is avascular
B.   consists of 35% protein
C.   is suspended by the zonule which inserts into the ciliary body
D.   the anterior capsule is responsible for the formation of new lens fibres
E.   is fully developed at birth

11. The meibomian glands:

A.   are suderiferous glands
B.   communicate with the eyelash follicles
C.   open anterior to the gray line
D.   contribute secretions to the deepest layer of the tear film
E.   number approximately 25 in each eyelid

12. The sclera:

A.   has the same histological structure as the cornea
B.   maximum thickness is approximately 1 mm
C.   is thinnest in the region of the insertion of the extraocular muscles
D.   is continuous with the lamina cribrosa
E.   the principal collagen is type I

13. **Bruch's membrane:**

A. its inner layer is the basement membrane of the retinal pigment epithelium
B. has 3 layers
C. is separated from the choroid by the suprachoroidal space
D. is continuous with the ciliary epithelium
E. has a central collagenous layer

14. **The ophthalmic artery:**

A. arises from the internal carotid artery within the cavernous sinus
B. usually passes superior to the optic nerve
C. the first intraorbital branch is the central retinal artery
D. communicates with branches of the external carotid artery
E. supplies all the orbital structures except the lacrimal gland

15. **The autonomic nervous system:**

A. the sympathetic nervous system supplies part of levator palpebrae superioris
B. the parasympathetic pathway to the pupil synapses in the ciliary ganglion
C. innervates the major retinal blood vessels
D. the supply to the lacrimal gland originates in the superior salivatory nucleus and exits the brainstem with the facial nerve
E. the sympathetic supply to the pupil originates in the Edinger–Westphal nucleus

16. Cerebral arteries:

A. the posterior cerebral arteries arise from the basilar artery
B. the middle cerebral arteries supply the optic tracts
C. the posterior cerebral arteries supply the optic radiations
D. the cranial nerve nuclei are supplied by the basilar and vertebral arteries
E. the optic chiasm is principally supplied by the middle cerebral arteries

17. The superior sagittal sinus:

A. contains arachnoid villi
B. is continuous with the sigmoid sinus
C. lies outside the dura
D. is joined by the inferior sagittal sinus
E. runs along the free edge of the falx cerebri

18. The fourth ventricle:

A. separates the pons from the cerebellum
B. communicates with the subarachnoid space via the foramen of Munro
C. its roof is partly formed by the superior medullary velum
D. does not contain choroid plexus
E. connects directly with the central canal of the spinal cord

19. The pituitary gland:

A.   the posterior lobe arises from the forebrain
B.   the anterior lobe arises from the foregut
C.   the pituitary stalk lies anterior to the optic chiasm
D.   lies outside the dura
E.   is connected to the hypothalamus by portal vessels

20. The primary visual cortex:

A.   lies either side of the calcarine sulcus
B.   is principally located on the lateral aspect of the occipital lobe
C.   is equivalent to the striate cortex
D.   has more layers than the rest of the cerebral cortex
E.   projects to the ipsilateral lateral geniculate nucleus

GENERAL PATHOLOGY, MICROBIOLOGY AND IMMUNOLOGY

21. Neonatal inclusion conjunctivitis:

A. is more common after Caesarian sections
B. is a viral infection
C. is best treated with topical tetracyclines
D. is often associated with genital infection in the neonate
E. is prevented by silver nitrate prophylaxis

22. Dysthyroid ophthalmopathy:

A. endocrine thyroid function is abnormal in all cases
B. the extraocular muscles most commonly involved are the inferior recti
C. ptosis is common
D. absence of thyroid antibodies indicates inactive disease
E. is synonymous with ophthalmic Graves' disease

23. Basal cell carcinoma:

A. frequently metastasises
B. may be multifocal
C. originates in the basal layers of the dermis
D. accounts for more than 90% of malignant eyelid tumours
E. medial canthal lesions have a good prognosis

24. Giant cell arteritis:

A.   the incidence is greatest in the 7th decade of life
B.   is rare before the age of 55
C.   its most common ocular presentation is anterior ischaemic optic neuropathy
D.   always causes an elevated ESR
E.   histological diagnosis requires the presence of giant cells on temporal artery biopsy

25. Neisseriae:

A.   are Gram-negative diplococci
B.   are always sensitive to penicillin
C.   are usually cultured on chocolate agar
D.   may colonise the pharynx
E.   characteristically cause a mildly purulent conjunctivitis

26. Acanthamoeba:

A.   is a free-living protozoan
B.   may be isolated from tapwater
C.   does not grow in culture at less than 37°C
D.   is usually sensitive to gentamicin
E.   has an encysted form

27. Myasthenia gravis:

A. is principally a disorder of acetylcholine production
B. may be associated with thymoma
C. does not respond to systemic steroid therapy
D. may be diagnosed by a trial of pyridostigmine
E. sensory loss is occasionally present

28. Choroidal malignant melanoma:

A. usually arises from a choroidal naevus
B. spindle cells are a poor prognostic sign
C. rarely spreads by the haematogenous route
D. is always darkly pigmented
E. peripapillary lesions have a poor prognosis

29. Vitamin A:

A. deficiency leads to conjunctival keratinisation
B. deficiency causes night blindness
C. is stored in the liver
D. toxicity may cause papilloedema
E. is derived from green vegetables

30. The following may be transmitted by X-linked inheritance:

A. retinitis pigmentosa
B. Duchenne muscular dystrophy
C. galactosaemia
D. Leber's hereditary optic neuropathy
E. dystrophia myotonica

OCULAR AND VISUAL PHYSIOLOGY

31. Vestibular eye movements:

A. are dependent upon VIIIth nerve function
B. are responsible for the doll's eye phenomenon
C. are responsible for caloric-induced nystagmus
D. the duration of post-rotatory nystagmus is increased in a blind patient
E. vestibular nystagmus has a pendular waveform

32. The electroretinogram (ERG):

A. the flash ERG is abnormal in macular disease
B. the cone ERG is elicited by slow flicker stimuli
C. the pattern ERG is a useful measure of visual acuity
D. uncorrected refractive errors may adversely affect the pattern ERG
E. the flash ERG normally contains oscillatory potentials

33. The pattern visual evoked response (VER):

A. is best recorded using a contact lens mounted electrode
B. the latency of the first major peak is normally 150 msec
C. may be used to diagnose chiasmal disease
D. is absent in functional blindness
E. does not depend upon normal retinal function

34. The pupillary light reflex:

A. an afferent pupillary defect does not occur in retinal disease
B. in Horner's syndrome redilatation after a light stimulus is prolonged
C. light near dissociation is a sign of midbrain disease
D. the direct and consensual responses to light are normally equal
E. is not present in the premature infant before 38 weeks' gestation

35. Intraocular pressure:

A. is usually at its highest level in the afternoon
B. is always less than the episcleral venous pressure
C. is increased in hydrocephalus
D. increases with age in Europeans
E. increases on Valsalva manoeuvre

36. Tears:

A. are present from birth
B. the results of Schirmer's test are increased by topical anaesthesia
C. basal tear secretion is produced by the palpebral lobe of the lacrimal gland
D. the tear film break-up time is an index of aqueous tear deficiency
E. have an alkaline pH

37. The lens:

A. the lens is kept relatively dehydrated by the action of the lens epithelium
B. glucose concentration is higher in the lens than the aqueous
C. transmission of ultraviolet light increases with age
D. lens fibres continue to be produced throughout life
E. the zonules are made of collagen

38. Visual acuity:

A. is a measure of minimum resolution
B. the forced choice preferential looking test cannot be used in children less than 2 years of age
C. the Sheridan–Gardner test is useful in dysphasia
D. the crowding phenomenon indicates an ability to see a lower line on the Snellen chart when lines of letters rather than single letters are viewed
E. each letter of the 6/6 Snellen line subtends an angle of 6° at 6 metres

39. Intraocular pressure:

A. the Goldmann tonometer is an indentation tonometer
B. may be decreased by increasing blood osmolarity
C. tonography is a measure of ciliary body function
D. scleral rigidity influences the calibration of the Schiotz tonometer
E. alignment of the prism during Goldmann tonometry should be adjusted according to the axis of corneal astigmatism

40. Perimetry:

A. a Bjerrum screen at 1 metre measures the central 30° of vision
B. suprathreshold perimetry is useful for screening for visual field defects
C. the Goldmann perimeter can only be used for kinetic perimetry
D. in automated perimetry visual fixation is assessed by repeated testing of the blind spot
E. in automated perimetry the background illumination is varied according to the testing programme

41. In the retina:

A. there are twice as many rods as cones
B. the central 10° does not contain any rods
C. rhodopsin is present in both rods and cones
D. visual pigments are absent in congenital achromatopsia
E. the luteal pigment is found only at the fovea centralis

42. Cornea:

A. the epithelium of the central cornea is supplied with oxygen by the limbal capillaries
B. the cornea is a barrier to ultraviolet radiation
C. transmission of light through the cornea is almost 100% throughout the visible spectrum
D. corneal thickness increases during prolonged eyelid closure
E. increased intraocular pressure produces epithelial oedema prior to development of stromal oedema

43. Aqueous humour:

A. is produced by passive diffusion
B. uveo–scleral outflow refers to a route of aqueous drainage via the suprachoroidal space
C. supplies oxygen and glucose to the lens and cornea
D. has the same protein concentration as plasma
E. 10% is absorbed by the iris stroma

44. Primary visual cortex:

A. the striae of Gennari correspond to layer IVB
B. all areas receive input from both eyes
C. corresponds to Brodmann Area 4
D. binocularly driven cells only respond to binocular stimulation
E. ocular dominance columns are restricted to layers III to VI

45. Eye movements:

A. maximum velocity of saccades is 700°/sec
B. saccadic eye movements are generated by the frontal eye fields
C. divergence is a purely passive phenomenon
D. vergence eye movements occur as a response to retinal disparity
E. convergence and accommodation cannot be dissociated

46. The pupil:

A. the pupillary light response pathway synapses in the lateral geniculate nucleus
B. the light response is mediated by the superior division of the third nerve
C. hippus indicates iris denervation
D. normally dilates to hydroxyamphetamine drops
E. normally constricts to 0.1% pilocarpine

47. Lids:

A. the muscles of the eyelid are supplied by both the VIIth and IIIrd cranial nerves
B. the blink reflex normally produces bilateral eyelid closure
C. forced lid closure is usually accompanied by downward deviation of the eyes
D. blinking does not involve the orbital portion of the orbicularis muscle
E. lid closure results in dilatation of the lacrimal sac

48. **Ocular motility:**

A.   the yoke muscle of the left medial rectus is the right medial rectus

B.   the superior oblique muscle produces intorsion when the eye is abducted

C.   the inferior oblique muscle attaches to the globe in the region of the macula

D.   Hering's law states that agonist and antagonist muscles receive equal innervation

E.   fusional amplitudes are a measure of heterophoria

49. **Binocular vision:**

A.   is dependent upon good visual acuity in each eye

B.   is not present until the 2nd year of life

C.   stereopsis is produced by simultaneous stimulation of corresponding retinal points

D.   depth perception requires binocular vision

E.   the angle kappa is normally positive

50. **Colour vision:**

A.   hue is dependent on the frequency of the ambient light

B.   green light has more energy than blue light

C.   opponent colour cells are maximally activated by white light

D.   the retina is not sensitive to electromagnetic radiation outside the visible spectrum

E.   the maximum sensitivity of the dark adapted eye is at a shorter wavelength than in the light-adapted eye

GENERAL PHARMACOLOGY, GENERAL PHYSIOLOGY AND BIOCHEMISTRY

51. Acetazolamide:

A.   is associated with aplastic anaemia
B.   increases CSF secretion
C.   may be administered topically to the eye
D.   is contraindicated in renal failure
E.   is chemically related to the sulphonamides

52. Adrenaline eye drops:

A.   are usually administered in a concentration of 0.1%
B.   cause cystoid macular oedema in the phakic eye
C.   may cause a cicatrising conjunctivitis
D.   are contraindicated in coronary artery disease
E.   should be stored in the dark

53. The following drugs may cause retinal damage:

A.   ethambutol
B.   chloroquine
C.   tamoxifen
D.   rifampicin
E.   digitalis

54. Insulin:

A.   decreases hepatic glucose output
B.   increases intracellular potassium
C.   increases uptake of amino-acids into skeletal muscle
D.   is produced by the exocrine pancreas
E.   the C-protein is cleaved prior to release and retained within the pancreatic cells

55. Haemoglobin:

A.   haemoglobin is still 95% saturated at an oxygen partial pressure of 80 mmHg
B.   glycosylated haemoglobin (HbA1c) is the product of an enzymatic process
C.   the abnormality in HbS is confined to a single amino acid substitution
D.   becomes more dissociated with increasing pH
E.   foetal haemoglobin has a lesser affinity for oxygen than adult haemoglobin

56. Arachidonic acid metabolism:

A.   arachidonic acid is derived from cell wall phospholipids
B.   the cyclo-oxygenase pathway produces prostaglandins
C.   phospholipase A is inhibited by corticosteroids
D.   leukotrienes are derivatives of prostaglandins
E.   aspirin inhibits production of prostaglandins and leukotrienes

57. β-Blockers:

A. betaxolol is a selective β_1 antagonist
B. β-blockers increase awareness of hypoglycaemia
C. selective β_1 antagonists have no effect on the bronchial tree
D. overdose is treated with intravenous glucagon
E. β-blockers do not cross the blood–brain barrier

58. Antimicrobial agents:

A. the most effective combination is a bacteriocidal agent together with a bacteriostatic agent
B. cephalosporins are frequently effective by mouth
C. ciprofloxacin is one of the recently produced penicillins
D. the aminoglycosides act by interfering with bacterial cell wall metabolism
E. nystatin is particularly effective against filamentous fungi

59. Atropine toxicity causes:

A. bradycardia
B. intestinal atony
C. cutaneous vasodilatation
D. restlessness
E. postural hypotension

60. The heart:

A. the sino-atrial node is regulated by a resting vagal tone
B. the QRS complex of the ECG is produced by depolarization spreading through the conducting system of the ventricles
C. the normal P–R interval is 0.2 sec
D. β-blockers decrease atrio-ventricular conduction
E. closure of the tricuspid valve is responsible for the a wave of the jugular pulse

CLINICAL SCIENCES

61. Epiphora:

A. in childhood the most common aetiology is congenital canalicular obstruction
B. is a frequent symptom of congenital glaucoma
C. in adults may resolve spontaneously due to decreased tear production
D. may be due to *Actinomyces canaliculitis*
E. may be associated with telecanthus

62. Mucocoeles:

A. should be treated before any intraocular surgery is undertaken
B. are associated with Le Fort type 1 facial fracture
C. may be due to herpes zoster infection
D. are usually treated with dacryocystectomy
E. acute bacterial infection requires incisional drainage

63. Lacrimal gland tumours:

A. adenocarcinomas are usually painless
B. can occur in the pluriglandular syndrome
C. erosion of the bony fossa indicates malignant disease
D. usually produce axial proptosis
E. anaesthesia over the lateral wall of the orbit is an indication of malignancy

64. Eyelid tumours:

A. basal cell carcinoma spreads by metastasis to the pre-auricular lymph nodes
B. basal cell carcinoma more commonly involves the upper lid
C. keratoacanthoma should be treated by wide excision
D. lymphatic spread of medial eyelid tumours is to the submental glands
E. meibomian gland carcinoma may present as a chronic blepharitis

65. Ptosis:

A. in levator dystrophy the degree of ptosis increases on downgaze
B. levator aponeurotic defects are associated with reduction of levator function
C. presence of a skin crease in congenital ptosis indicates good levator function
D. the ptosis of myasthenia gravis is often absent upon waking
E. the Fasanella–Servat procedure is only useful in mild degrees of ptosis

66. Lid malposition:

A. upper lid entropion results in dystichiasis
B. facial nerve palsy results in entropion
C. upper lid entropion is usually cicatricial
D. lower lid ectropion occurs in Horner's syndrome
E. lid laxity is the major factor predisposing to senile ectropion

67. Blepharospasm:

A. is usually bilateral
B. may spread to involve the lower face and platysma
C. may be treated by botulinum toxin injections to the levator muscle
D. may be a manifestation of extrapyramidal disease
E. is often associated with ocular surface disorders

68. Dysthyroid eye disease:

A. lid retraction and lid lag are early clinical signs
B. is the most common cause of unilateral axial proptosis
C. is associated with superior limbic kerato-conjunctivitis
D. most commonly affects the superior rectus muscle
E. extraocular muscle enlargement involves the muscle tendon

69. Carotico-cavernous fistula:

A.   is usually spontaneous in young people
B.   may present with a VIth nerve palsy
C.   usually produces an orbital bruit
D.   results in arterialisation of the conjunctival veins
E.   often resolves spontaneously in elderly patients

70. Orbital pseudotumour (idiopathic orbital inflammation):

A.   may present with a ptosis
B.   is usually painless
C.   may present with isolated lacrimal gland enlargement
D.   50% of cases are associated with systemic lymphoma
E.   is not usually steroid responsive

71. Orbital cellulitis:

A.   requires a full 5-day course of oral antibiotics
B.   is usually secondary to frontal sinus disease
C.   causes non-axial proptosis
D.   restricted ocular motility indicates cavernous sinus thrombosis
E.   nasal swabs are the most useful method of identifying the causative organism

72. Viral conjunctivitis:

A. epidemic keratoconjunctivitis is caused by a coxsackie virus
B. usually causes a purulent conjunctival discharge
C. adenovirus infection usually resolves within 1 week
D. pre-auricular lymphadenopathy is a feature of adenovirus infection
E. herpetic conjunctivitis is often associated with a blepharitis

73. Keratoconus:

A. is most frequently managed with soft contact lenses
B. is usually unilateral
C. is inherited as an autosomal dominant trait
D. acute hydrops may lead to corneal rupture
E. is associated with Haab's striae

74. Fuchs' endothelial dystrophy:

A. is usually bilateral
B. is characterised by central corneal guttata
C. is more common in females
D. initially causes stromal thickening
E. is characterised by blurring of vision that increases during the day

75. Corneal degenerations and dystrophies:

A.   calcium is a major component of band keratopathy
B.   Salzmann's nodular dystrophy is frequently seen in trachoma
C.   macular dystrophy is autosomal recessive
D.   in corneal arcus the lipid deposition is principally in the mid-stroma
E.   map dot fingerprint dystrophy causes recurrent corneal erosions

76. Acanthamoeba keratitis:

A.   rarely occurs in contact lens wearers
B.   infection usually begins at the limbus
C.   is usually painless
D.   the organism will grow on blood agar
E.   is usually associated with a hypopyon

77. Herpetic keratitis:

A.   primarily manifests as a dendritic ulcer
B.   epithelial disease leads to corneal scarring
C.   is associated with decreased corneal sensation
D.   rarely causes corneal perforation
E.   bilateral disease is a feature of atopy

78. Posterior scleritis:

A. is usually painless
B. causes proptosis
C. can be diagnosed on an ultrasound scan
D. causes macular oedema
E. necessitates systemic steroid treatment

79. Episcleritis:

A. causes scleral swelling
B. may produce a peripheral ulcerative keratitis
C. often resolves spontaneously
D. is responsive to non-steroidal anti-inflammatory drugs
E. occurs in Reiter's disease

80. Cataracts:

A. sunflower cataracts occur in Wilson's disease
B. propeller cataracts occur in atopic dermatitis
C. presenile cataracts occur in neurofibromatosis type 1
D. christmas tree cataracts occur in myotonic dystrophy
E. galactosaemic cataracts are usually present at birth

81. Primary open-angle glaucoma:

A.   affects 5% of the British population
B.   is more common in diabetics
C.   is less common in myopes
D.   is more severe in blacks than whites
E.   there are characteristic histological changes in the trabecular
      meshwork

82. Secondary glaucoma:

A.   pigmentary glaucoma most commonly affects young adult
      myopes
B.   in pigmentary glaucoma exercise may induce marked elevation of
      intraocular pressure
C.   pseudoexfoliative glaucoma is more common amongst blacks
D.   pseudoexfoliative glaucoma predisposes to zonular rupture and
      vitreous loss during cataract surgery
E.   increased angle pigmentation is a feature of pseudoexfoliative
      glaucoma

83. Steroid-induced elevation of intraocular pressure:

A.   only occurs with topical steroids
B.   is always reversible with discontinuation of steroid therapy
C.   is more common in patients with primary open-angle glaucoma
D.   is not dependent on the potency of steroids administered
E.   is an inherited trait

84. **Laser surgery for glaucoma:**

A.   laser trabeculoplasty can be performed with the diode laser
B.   laser trabeculoplasty is more effective in eyes with greater angle pigmentation
C.   YAG laser iridotomy is easier to perform in blue rather than brown irides
D.   argon laser iridotomy is easier to perform in blue rather than brown irides
E.   the Abrahams lens is used for laser trabeculoplasty

85. **Glaucoma therapy:**

A.   selective β_1 antagonists are more effective than non-selective agents
B.   propine causes less intraocular side-effects than adrenaline
C.   the maximum useful concentration of pilocarpine is 4%
D.   pilocarpine is contraindicated in uveitis
E.   parasympathomimetic agents are not effective in aphakes

86. **Neovascular glaucoma is associated with:**

A.   choroidal melanoma
B.   carotid artery occlusion
C.   branch retinal artery occlusion
D.   posterior uveitis
E.   carotico-cavernous fistula

87. Acute anterior uveitis is associated with:

A. Reiter's disease
B. secondary syphilis
C. presumed ocular histoplasmosis syndrome (POHS)
D. relapsing polychondritis
E. ankylosing spondylitis

88. Pars planitis:

A. usually presents over the age of 40
B. produces a red eye
C. visual loss is most often due to vitritis
D. is usually unilateral
E. periocular steroids are contraindicated

89. Toxoplasmic retino-choroiditis:

A. rarely affects the posterior pole
B. rarely causes significant vitritis
C. treatment is capable of eradicating the organism
D. is always due to congenital infection
E. may resolve spontaneously

90. **Acquired immunodeficiency syndrome (AIDS):**

A. cytomegalovirus retinitis does not respond to foscarnet therapy
B. cotton-wool spots do not indicate opportunistic infection of the retina
C. may be transmitted by corneal transplantation
D. results in low CD-4 T-cell counts
E. HIV-1 infection predisposes to herpes zoster ophthalmicus

91. **Sympathetic ophthalmia:**

A. does not occur after intraocular surgery
B. Dahlen–Fuchs nodules occur on the iris
C. causes optic disc swelling
D. rarely causes recurrent episodes of inflammation
E. inflammatory cells in the retrolenticular space is an early clinical sign

92. **Behçet's disease:**

A. rarely leads to blindness
B. branch retinal artery occlusions are a common finding
C. is particularly common in Japan
D. is associated with vena caval thrombosis
E. is characterised by oro-genital ulceration

93. Sarcoidosis:

A. Busacca nodules occur on the iris margin
B. ocular involvement occurs in less than 5% of patients
C. the Kveim test involves intradermal injection of an extract of human splenic tissue
D. the characteristic histopathological finding is caseating granulomas
E. hilar lymphadenopathy on chest X-ray is usually associated with pulmonary symptoms

94. Fuchs' heterochromic cyclitis:

A. cataract is uncommon
B. the keratitic precipitates disappear with topical steroid therapy
C. posterior synechiae do not occur
D. may cause a vitritis
E. is associated with abnormal blood vessels in the anterior chamber angle

95. Vitreous haemorrhage may be due to:

A. background diabetic retinopathy
B. Eales' disease
C. disciform macular degeneration
D. posterior vitreous detachment
E. subarachnoid haemorrhage

96. **In retinitis pigmentosa:**

A. X-linked recessive inheritance is associated with the most rapidly progressive disease
B. the earliest field loss is a generalised constriction
C. ERG abnormalities precede visual field loss
D. nyctalopia is a late feature
E. loss of visual acuity may be due to posterior subcapsular cataract

97. **Central retinal vein occlusion:**

A. is more common in diabetes mellitus
B. has an increased incidence in primary open-angle glaucoma
C. is complicated by neovascular glaucoma in 20% of untreated cases
D. is a complication of carotid artery disease
E. a relative afferent pupillary defect is suggestive of an ischaemic central retinal vein occlusion

98. **Sickle cell retinopathy:**

A. is most severe in the SS genotype
B. causes sea-fan vascular proliferation
C. rarely causes optic disc neovascularization
D. is associated with angioid streaks
E. retinal photocoagulation does not influence the final visual outcome

99. Diabetic retinopathy:

A. proliferative retinopathy only occurs in insulin-dependent diabetes
B. less than 5% of patients with ischaemic maculopathy will develop proliferative retinopathy within 2 years
C. pan-retinal photocoagulation may exacerbate macular oedema
D. intra-retinal microvascular anomalies (IRMAs) are a feature of pre-proliferative retinopathy
E. is common amongst patients from the Indian subcontinent

100. Retinal artery occlusion:

A. central retinal artery occlusion is complicated by neovascular glaucoma in less than 5% of cases
B. branch retinal artery occlusion is rarely caused by emboli
C. branch retinal artery occlusion is a feature of giant cell arteritis
D. central retinal artery occlusion causes optic disc haemorrhages
E. central retinal artery occlusion is a complication of subacute bacterial endocarditis

101. Haematological disorders:

A. white-centered retinal haemorrhages occur in leukaemia
B. polycythaemia causes dilatation of the retinal veins
C. acute blood loss may lead to ischaemic optic neuropathy
D. megaloblastic anaemia is associated with optic atrophy
E. sickle cell disease increases the risks of anterior segment ischaemia after squint surgery

102. Retinal vascular disease:

A. Coat's disease causes subretinal exudation
B. Eales' disease is associated with recurrent vitreous haemorrhages
C. retinal macroaneurysms are more common in females
D. Eales' disease is usually unilateral
E. retinal macroaneurysms rarely thrombose spontaneously

103. Central serous retinopathy:

A. is more common in men than women
B. produces no abnormality on fluorescein angiography
C. rarely resolves spontaneously
D. is often complicated by choroidal neovascularization
E. visual acuity is frequently improved by a hypermetropic correction

104. 'Bull's eye' maculopathy occurs in:

A. chloroquine toxicity
B. Tay–Sachs disease
C. neurofibromatosis type 1
D. cone dystrophy
E. Laurence–Moon–Biedl syndrome

105. Cystoid macular oedema:

A.   causes a 'flower petal' appearance on fluorescein angiography
B.   is associated with vitreous loss during cataract surgery
C.   is a complication of retinitis pigmentosa
D.   is the major cause of visual loss in pars planitis
E.   indicates macular ischaemia when seen in association with diabetic retinopathy

106. Pigment epithelial detachments:

A.   are associated with choroidal neovascularization
B.   are more clearly demarcated on fluorescein angiography than serous retinal detachments
C.   may be haemorrhagic
D.   usually occur outside the retinal vascular arcades
E.   indicate a breakdown of the inner blood–retinal barrier

107. The following predispose to sub-retinal neovascularization:

A.   angioid streaks
B.   optic nerve head drusen
C.   full thickness macular hole
D.   diabetic retinopathy
E.   macular branch retinal vein occlusion

108. Electrodiagnostics:

A. the pattern ERG assesses the function of the peripheral retina
B. the EOG is measured with a flash stimulus
C. the pattern VER may be used to assess retinal function in the presence of opaque media
D. the EOG may be used to measure saccadic eye movements
E. the flash VER is normal in retinitis pigmentosa

109. Macular function tests:

A. the macular photostress test is a measure of retinal photoreceptor pigment regeneration
B. neutral density filters reduce the visual acuity less severely in amblyopia than in macular disease
C. the Maddox rod test requires clear media
D. the Amsler grid at reading distance tests the central 20° of vision
E. the Pulfrich phenomenon is a feature of unilateral macular disease

110. Choroidal malignant melanoma:

A. is rarely associated with serous retinal detachment
B. spindle cells indicate a good prognosis
C. haematogenous spread is the commonest route of metastasis
D. choroidal excavation is seen on ultrasound scanning
E. transillumination of the globe is used to localize the lesion at the time of surgery

111. Acute retrobulbar optic neuritis is usually associated with:

A. pain on eye movements
B. a swollen optic disc
C. fluorescein leakage from the optic disc
D. altitudinal field defect
E. normal pupillary reactions

112. Non-arteritic anterior ischaemic optic neuropathy:

A. usually causes an inferior altitudinal field defect
B. is associated with a raised ESR
C. visual loss usually develops over 2–3 days
D. visual acuity usually improves with time
E. there is no leakage from the optic disc on fluorescein angiography

113. Papilloedema:

A. is usually associated with loss of colour vision
B. spontaneous retinal venous pulsation is characteristically present
C. the optic cup is obliterated early in the development of the disc swelling
D. disc haemorrhages indicate chronic disc swelling
E. is associated with visual obscurations

114. **Childhood esotropia:**

A. in congenital esotropia the esodeviation is usually greater for near than for distance
B. congenital esotropia is associated with latent nystagmus
C. fully accommodative esotropia is associated with good binocular function
D. patients with fully accommodative esotropia usually require squint surgery
E. convergence excess esotropia can be treated with executive bifocal spectacles

115. **Incomitant squints:**

A. in superior oblique palsy the hyperdeviation is greater on gaze to the ipsilateral side
B. pupillary involvement in a third nerve palsy suggests a compressive lesion
C. in sixth nerve palsy the esodeviation is greater for near than for distance
D. Brown's syndrome causes restriction of elevation in adduction
E. Duane's retraction syndrome usually results in a head turn towards the affected side

116. **Pupils:**

A. a relative afferent pupillary defect cannot be detected in the presence of a unilateral total third nerve palsy
B. optic nerve compression causes pupillary dilatation
C. 0.1% pilocarpine will constrict a Holmes–Adie pupil
D. cocaine is used to differentiate pre-ganglionic from a post-ganglionic Horner's syndrome
E. a small pupil in the presence of a third nerve palsy indicates a lesion in the cavernous sinus

117. Suprasellar masses causing chiasmal compression:

A. optic atrophy is an early sign
B. may produce diplopia in the absence of cranial nerve palsy
C. are often associated with papilloedema
D. in a child calcification suggests craniopharyngioma
E. bitemporal hemianopias always involve the peripheral visual fields

118. Retinopathy of prematurity:

A. is not present at birth
B. predominantly involves the nasal peripheral retina
C. 10% phenylephrine is used for pupillary dilatation for fundal examination
D. 'plus' disease refers to vascular changes in the posterior segment
E. retinal cryotherapy is recommended for stage 5 disease

119. Paediatric ophthalmology:

A. familial retinoblastoma may be present within the first 2 months of life
B. ocular albinism is autosomal dominant
C. optic nerve hypoplasia is associated with diabetes insipidus
D. delayed visual maturation is associated with an abnormal ERG
E. Leber's congenital amaurosis is a retinal dystrophy

120. Blindness:

A. the World Health Organisation's definition of blindness is visual acuity of worse than 3/60 in the better eye

B. the World Health Organisation estimates that there are over 40 million people in the world with vision 6/60 or worse in each eye

C. cataract is the commonest cause of blindness worldwide

D. in the United Kingdom it is suggested that to be eligible for partially sighted registration a patient should have a visual acuity of 6/60 or worse in the better eye

E. in England and Wales the commonest cause of newly-registered blindness amongst adults over 65 is macular degeneration

Answers

1.
A – **F** the lens capsule is derived from surface ectoderm
B – **T** the ciliary muscle is derived from neural crest ectoderm
C – **T**
D – **F** levator palpebrae superioris and the extraocular muscles are derived from embryonic mesoderm
E – **T**

2.
A – **T**
B – **F** the sixth nerve nucleus is in the pons
C – **T**
D – **T**
E – **F** the lateral geniculate nucleus is in the thalamus

3.
A – **F** the ophthalmic artery passes through the optic foramen
B – **T**
C – **T**
D – **T**
E – **T**

4.
A – **F** the corneal epithelium is a stratified epithelium
B – **T**
C – **F** the cells of the corneal stroma are the keratocytes
D – **T**
E – **F** the corneal curvature determines the eye's refractive power

5.

A – T

B – F   the optic nerve meninges have the same structure as the
cerebral meninges

C – T

D – F   the laminar portion of the optic nerve is supplied by branches
of the short posterior ciliary arteries

E – T

6.

A – T

B – T

C – F   the medial wall of the orbit normally is convex with respect to
the globe

D – T

E – T

7.

A – F   the retina is thinnest at the fovea and thickest in the area of
the arcuate nerve fibre bundles

B – T

C – F   retinal vascularization is not completed until the 9th month of
gestation

D – T

E – F   the Müller cells extend from the internal to the external
limiting membranes

8.

A – T

B – T

C – T

D – F   levator palpebrae superioris is supplied by the superior
division of the oculomotor nerve

E – T

9.

A – **T**

B – **F**   the anterior cranial fossa contains the frontal lobes of the cerebrum

C – **T**

D – **T**

E – **F**   the lateral wall of the orbit lies outside the cranial cavity

10.

A – **T**

B – **T**

C – **T**

D – **F**   the anterior lens epithelium beneath the anterior capsule is responsible for the formation of new lens fibres

E – **F**   the lens continues to grow throughout life

11.

A – **F**   the meibomian glands are modified sebaceous glands

B – **F**   the meibomian glands do not communicate with the eyelash follicles

C – **F**   the meibomian glands open posterior to the gray line

D – **F**   the meibomian glands contribute secretions to the most superficial layer of the tear film

E – **T**

12.

A – **T**

B – **T**

C – **T**

D – **T**

E – **T**

13.

A – **T**

B – **F**   there are 5 layers

C – **F**   the suprachoroidal space lies external to the choroid

D – **F**   the layers of the ciliary epithelium are continuations of the retina and retinal pigment epithelium

E – **F**   Bruch's membrane has a central elastic layer

14.

A – **F**   the ophthalmic artery arises from the internal carotid within the cranial cavity

B – **F**   the ophthalmic artery usually passes inferior to the optic nerve

C – **T**

D – **T**

E – **F**   the ophthalmic artery supplies all the orbital structures including the lacrimal gland

15.

A – **T**

B – **T**

C – **F**   the major retinal blood vessels have no nervous supply

D – **T**

E – **F**   the Edinger–Westphal nucleus is the origin of the parasympathetic supply to the pupil

16.

A – **T**

B – **T**

C – **F**   the optic radiations are supplied by the middle cerebral arteries

D – **T**

E – **F**   the optic chiasm receives no supply from the middle cerebral arteries

17.

A – **T**
B – **F**   the superior sagittal sinus is continuous with the lateral (transverse) sinus
C – **F**   the superior sagittal sinus lies within the dura
D – **F**   the inferior sagittal sinus is continuous with the straight sinus
E – **F**   the superior sagittal sinus runs in the attached margin of the falx cerebri

18.

A – **T**
B – **F**   the fourth ventricle communicates with the subarachnoid space via the foramina of Magendie and Luschka
C – **T**
D – **F**   the fourth ventricle does contain choroid plexus
E – **T**

19.

A – **T**
B – **T**
C – **F**   the pituitary stalk lies posterior to the optic chiasm
D – **F**   the pituitary gland lies within the dura
E – **T**

20.

A – **T**
B – **F**   the primary visual cortex is principally located on the medial aspect of the occipital lobe
C – **T**
D – **F**   the primary visual cortex has the same number of layers as the rest of the cerebral cortex
E – **T**   as well as geniculo-striate projections there are also projections from the striate cortex back to the lateral geniculate nucleus

21.
A – **F**   neonatal inclusion conjunctivitis is acquired during vaginal delivery

B – **F**   neonatal inclusion conjunctivitis is caused by *Chlamydia trachomatis* which is an intracellular bacterium

C – **F**   systemic therapy is required and erythromycin is the agent of choice because of the side-effects from tetracyclines in children

D – **F**   adult inclusion conjunctivitis is associated with genital infection

E – **F**   silver nitrate is not effective against *Chlamydia*

22.
A – **F**   up to 10% of patients have normal thyroid endocrine function

B – **T**

C – **F**   ptosis is uncommon and usually indicates coincidental myasthenia gravis

D – **F**   there is no direct correlation between the presence or absence of thyroid antibodies and disease activity

E – **F**   ophthalmic Graves' disease is dysthyroid ophthalmopathy in the absence of thyroid endocrine dysfunction

23.
A – **F**   basal cell carcinoma very rarely metastasises

B – **T**

C – **F**   basal cell carcinoma originates in the basal layers of the epidermis

D – **T**

E – **F**   medial canthal lesions have a poor prognosis

24.

A – **F**   the incidence increases with increasing age beyond the 7th decade of life

B – **T**

C – **T**

D – **F**   the ESR may be normal

E – **F**   although they are diagnostic, giant cells are not always present, and diagnosis is often based upon finding a lymphocytic infiltration of the vessel wall with fragmentation of the internal elastic lamina

25.

A – **T**

B – **F**   penicillin resistant Neisseriae are increasingly common

C – **T**

D – **T**

E – **F**   conjunctivitis due to Neisseriae characteristically causes a markedly purulent discharge

26.

A – **T**

B – **T**

C – **F**   some strains will grow better at 25°C than 37°C

D – **F**   *Acanthamoeba* is not sensitive to gentamicin

E – **T**

27.

A – **F**   the principal abnormality is the presence of antibodies to the post-synaptic acetylcholine receptor

B – **T**   thymoma occurs in about 10% of cases

C – **F**   systemic steroids are often effective

D – **T**

E – **F**   sensory loss does not occur in myasthenia

28.
A – **F** choroidal malignant melanoma uncommonly arises from a choroidal naevus

B – **F** spindle cells are a good prognostic sign

C – **F** choroidal malignant melanoma usually spreads by the haematogenous route

D – **F** choroidal malignant melanoma may be amelanotic

E – **T**

29.
A – **T**

B – **T**

C – **T**

D – **T**

E – **T**

30.
A – **T**

B – **T**

C – **F** galactosaemia is autosomal recessive

D – **F** Leber's hereditary optic neuropathy is transmitted by mitochondrial inheritance

E – **F** dystrophia myotonica is autosomal dominant

31.
A – **T**

B – **T**

C – **T**

D – **T** dampening of post-rotatory nystagmus is increased by visual fixation

E – **F** vestibular nystagmus is a jerk nystagmus

32.

A – **F** in macular disease the flash ERG is normal but the pattern ERG may be abnormal

B – **F** the cone ERG is elicited by fast flicker stimuli

C – **F** the pattern VEP provides an approximate measure of visual acuity

D – **T** any response to a pattern stimulus may be affected by uncorrected refractive errors

E – **T**

33.

A – **F** a contact lens mounted electrode is not required but scalp electrodes are used

B – **F** the latency is normally about 100 msec

C – **T** hemifield stimuli can be used to assess chiasmal function

D – **F** the pattern VER is present in functional blindness

E – **F** the VER is dependent upon normal retinal function

34.

A – **F** extensive retinal disease will cause an afferent pupillary defect

B – **T** a characteristic sign in Horner's syndrome is the redilatation lag

C – **T**

D – **T**

E – **F** the pupillary light response first becomes apparent at 29 weeks' gestation

35.

A – **F** intraocular pressure is usually maximal during the morning

B – **T**

C – **F** intraocular pressure is not related to CSF pressure

D – **T** in Europeans intraocular pressure increases with age whereas in the Japanese it falls with age

E – **T**

36.

A – **T**

B – **T**

C – **F** basal tear secretion is produced by the accessory lacrimal glands

D – **F** the tear film break-up time correlates with mucin deficiency and not with aqueous tear deficiency

E – **T**

37.

A – **T**

B – **F** glucose concentration is 5 times lower in the lens than in the aqueous

C – **F** transmission of ultraviolet light decreases with age

D – **T**

E – **F** the zonules are made of non-collagenous protein

38.

A – **F** visual acuity is a measure of maximum resolution

B – **F** the forced choice preferential looking test can be used in young babies

C – **T**

D – **F** the crowding phenomenon indicates an ability to see a lower line on the Snellen chart when single letters rather than lines of letters are viewed

E – **F** each letter of the 6/6 Snellen line subtends an angle of 5 minutes of arc at 6 metres

39.

A – **F** the Goldmann tonometer is an applanation tonometer

B – **T**

C – **F** tonography is a measure of aqueous outflow

D – **T**

E – **T** the markings on the tip of the Goldmann tonometer facilitate the appropriate alignment

40.

A – **T**

B – **T**

C – **F**   both static and kinetic perimetry can be performed with the Goldmann perimeter

D – **T**

E – **F**   whenever possible the background illumination is standardised and kept constant in all forms of perimetry

41.

A – **F**   there are at least 10 times more rods than cones

B – **F**   rods are absent only in the central 1°

C – **F**   rhodopsin is confined to the rods

D – **F**   there is always at least one visual pigment present in congenital achromatopsia

E – **F**   luteal pigment is present throughout the macula

42.

A – **F**   the epithelium of the central cornea is supplied with oxygen by the tear film

B – **T**

C – **T**

D – **T**

E – **T**

43.

A – **F**   aqueous production depends upon ultrafiltration and active secretion

B – **T**

C – **T**   although the oxygen requirement of the lens is extremely small

D – **F**   aqueous has a lower protein concentration than plasma

E – **F**   water diffuses from the iris stroma into the aqueous

44.

A – T
B – F   the anterior extent of the primary visual cortex receives input from the far temporal field (temporal crescent) of the contralateral eye only
C – F   the primary visual cortex corresponds to Brodmann Area 17
D – F   binocularly driven cells respond to stimuli from either eye
E – F   ocular dominance columns extend throughout all layers of the primary visual cortex

45.

A – T
B – T
C – F   divergence is an active process, although the neural pathways are not yet fully defined
D – T
E – F   convergence and accommodation can be dissociated with prisms or minus lenses

46.

A – F   the pupillary light response fibres pass to the midbrain before reaching the lateral geniculate nucleus
B – F   the parasympathetic supply to the iris passes in the inferior division of the third nerve
C – F   hippus is physiological but in iris denervation it may be more marked
D – T   but in a post-ganglionic Horner's syndrome the pupil will not dilate to hydroxyamphetamine
E – F   pupillary constriction to 0.1% pilocarpine indicates denervation hypersensitivity

47.

A – **T**

B – **T**

C – **F** forced lid closure is usually accompanied by upward deviation of the eyes

D – **T**

E – **T**

48.

A – **F** the yoke muscle of the left medial rectus is the right lateral rectus

B – **T**

C – **T**

D – **T**

E – **F** fusional amplitudes are a measure of the maximum degree of retinal disparity that can be overcome by vergence movements, whereas heterophoria is a measure of the deviation that occurs when binocular function is disrupted

49.

A – **F** binocular vision may still be present when visual acuities are markedly reduced

B – **F** binocular vision is certainly present during the first year of life

C – **F** steropsis is produced by simultaneous stimulation of non-corresponding retinal points

D – **F** depth perception can be achieved with monocular clues

E – **T**

50.

A – **T**

B – **F** green light has less energy than blue light

C – **F** opponent colour cells are minimally activated by white light

D – **F** the retina is sensitive to electromagnetic radiation outside the visible spectrum but such stimuli are inadequate to form a visual image

E – **T** the maximum sensitivity of the dark adapted eye is at 510 nm and of the light-adapted eye is at 555 nm

51.
A – **T**
B – **F**   acetazolamide decreases CSF secretion
C – **F**   acetazolamide cannot be used topically but related
compounds are being studied for topical administration
D – **T**
E – **T**

52.
A – **F**   adrenaline eye drops are usually administered in a
concentration of 1.0%
B – **F**   cystoid macular oedema may be produced in the aphakic eye
C – **T**
D – **T**
E – **T**

53.
A – **F**   ethambutol may cause optic nerve damage
B – **T**
C – **T**
D – **F**   rifampicin may cause optic nerve disease
E – **T**

54.
A – **T**
B – **T**
C – **T**
D – **F**   insulin is produced by the endocrine pancreas
E – **F**   the C-protein is cleaved prior to release but is then released
into the bloodstream

55.

A – T
B – F   glycosylated haemoglobin (HbA1c) is the product of a
non-enzymatic process
C – T
D – F   increasing pH increases the oxygen affinity of haemoglobin
E – F   foetal haemoglobin has a greater affinity for oxygen than
adult haemoglobin

56.

A – T
B – T
C – T
D – F   leukotrienes are produced by the lipoxygenase pathway
E – F   aspirin only inhibits production of prostaglandins

57.

A – T
B – F β-blockers decrease awareness of hypoglycaemia
C – F   selective β_1-antagonists have relatively little effect on the
bronchial tree
D – T   glucagon is an inotrope that acts at a different receptor site
than β-blockers
E – F   certain β-blockers are able to cross the blood–brain barrier
and cause CNS side-effects

58.

A – F   a bacteriocidal agent and a bacteriostatic agent should not be
used in combination
B – F   very few cephalosporins are absorbed after oral
administration
C – F   ciprofloxacin is a quinolone
D – F   the aminoglycosides act by interfering with bacterial protein
metabolism
E – F   nystatin is relatively ineffective against filamentous fungi

59.

A – **F**   tachycardia
B – **T**
C – **T**
D – **T**
E – **F**

60.

A – **T**
B – **F**   the QRS complex of the ECG is produced by depolarization
              spreading through muscle of the ventricles
C – **F**   the normal P–R interval is 0.12–0.2 sec
D – **T**
E – **F**   atrial systole is responsible for the a wave of the jugular pulse

61.

A – **F**   childhood epiphora is usually due to delayed perforation of
              the lower end of the nasolacrimal duct
B – **T**
C – **T**
D – **T**
E – **T**   lacrimal drainage abnormalities are a common feature of
              cranio-facial anomalies

62.

A – **T**   because of the risk of endophthalmitis
B – **F**   Le Fort type 1 fractures involve the lower part of the
              mid-facial skeleton only
C – **F**   herpes zoster infection does not result in nasolacrimal duct
              obstruction
D – **F**   mucocoeles are usually treated by dacryocystorhinostomy.
              Dacryocystectomy may be indicated if dacryocystorhinostomy
              is unsuccessful or if there has been recurrent acute
              dacryocystitis
E – **F**   incisional drainage of acute dacryocystitis may lead to fistula
              formation

63.

A – **F** adenocarcinomas are usually painful

B – **F** the pluriglandular syndrome is an abnormality of endocrine glands

C – **T**

D – **F** the proptosis is usually non-axial with downward and inward displacement

E – **T**

64.

A – **F** spread of basal cell carcinoma is by local infiltration

B – **F** basal cell carcinoma more commonly affects the lower than the upper eyelid

C – **F** keratoacanthoma is a benign lesion which usually resolves spontaneously

D – **T**

E – **T**

65.

A – **F** in levator dystrophy the levator does not relax such that the ptosis becomes less marked on downgaze

B – **F** levator function is normal in levator aponeurotic defects

C – **T**

D – **T**

E – **T**

66.

A – **F** dystichiasis is eyelashes arising in an abnormal site and is not the result of entropion

B – **F** facial nerve palsy results in ectropion

C – **T**

D – **F** Horner's syndrome results in lower lid retraction

E – **T**

67.

A – **T**
B – **T**
C – **F**   botulinum toxin is injected into the orbicularis oculi muscles
D – **T**
E – **T**

68.

A – **T**
B – **T**
C – **T**
D – **F**   the inferior rectus is the most commonly affected extraocular muscle
E – **F**   extraocular muscle enlargement characteristically spares the muscle tendon

69.

A – **F**   in young people carotico-cavernous fistula is usually traumatic
B – **T**
C – **F**   although an orbital bruit is a characteristic sign of carotico-cavernous fistula it is relatively unusual
D – **T**
E – **T**

70.

A – **T**
B – **F**   orbital pseudotumour is usually painful
C – **T**
D – **F**   systemic lymphoma occurs in less than 5% of patients with orbital pseudotumour
E – **F**   orbital pseudotumour is usually steroid responsive

71.

A – F   orbital cellulitis requires parenteral therapy

B – F   orbital cellulitis is usually due to ethmoidal sinus disease

C – F   orbital cellulitis causes axial proptosis. The development of non-axial proptosis indicates abscess formation

D – F   restricted ocular motility is a feature of uncomplicated orbital cellulitis; it is restricted ocular motility in the fellow eye that indicates cavernous sinus thrombosis

E – F   blood cultures are more likely to identify the causative organism than nasal swabs

72.

A – F   epidemic keratoconjunctivitis is caused by an adenovirus

B – F   viral conjunctivitis causes a mucoid conjunctival discharge unless there is pseudo-membranous or membranous conjunctivitis

C – F   adenovirus infection usually persists for a number of weeks

D – T

E – T

73.

A – F   keratoconus is most frequently managed with rigid contact lenses

B – F   keratoconus is almost always bilateral

C – F   keratoconus is usually sporadic

D – F   corneal rupture is not a feature of acute hydrops

E – T

74.

A – T

B – T

C – T

D – F   the initial changes are in the endothelium

E – F   the visual blurring is maximal upon waking

75.

A – **T**
B – **T**
C – **T**
D – **T**
E – **T**

76.

A – **F**   it occurs most commonly in contact lens wearers
B – **F**   infection usually begins in the central cornea
C – **F**   it is usually painful
D – **F**   culture of the organism requires special media of a
         non-nutrient agar plate covered with a lawn of killed bacteria,
         usually *E. coli*
E – **F**   hypopyon formation suggests additional bacterial infection

77.

A – **T**
B – **F**   epithelial herpetic keratitis does not cause corneal scarring
C – **T**
D – **T**
E – **T**

78.

A – **F**   posterior scleritis is usually painful
B – **T**
C – **T**   A-scan ultrasound demonstrates the thickened sclera
D – **T**
E – **F**   posterior scleritis may respond to non-steroidal
         anti-inflammatory drugs just like anterior scleritis

79.

A – **F** scleral swelling indicates scleritis
B – **F** peripheral ulcerative keratitis occurs in scleritis but not in episcleritis
C – **T**
D – **T**
E – **T**

80.

A – **T**
B – **F** propeller cataracts occur in Fabry's disease
C – **F** presenile cataracts occur in neurofibromatosis type 2 not type 1
D – **T**
E – **F** galactosaemic cataracts usually develop after birth once the baby is exposed to dietary lactose

81.

A – **F** 0.5–1.0% of the over-40s
B – **T**
C – **F** it is more common in myopes
D – **T**
E – **F** the trabecular meshwork does not show changes other than those associated with ageing

82.

A – **T**
B – **T** exercise may produce a sudden increase in pigment liberation
C – **F** pseudoexfoliative glaucoma is more common in Northern Europeans
D – **T**
E – **T**

83.

A – **F**   it may occur with systemic administration or even topical application to the skin

B – **F**   the glaucoma may persist permanently after discontinuation of the steroids

C – **T**

D – **F**   there is a clear relationship to potency of the steroid administered

E – **T**   there is a clear familial predisposition

84.

A – **T**

B – **T**

C – **T**   blue irides are thinner than brown irides

D – **F**   the argon laser is dependent upon the presence of pigment for its efficacy

E – **F**   the Abraham lens is for peripheral iridotomy

85.

A – **F**   non-selective agents tend to be more effective than β_1-selective agents

B – **F**   propine causes less extraocular side-effects but the same intraocular side-effects as adrenaline

C – **F**   in pigmented eyes concentrations of pilocarpine of up to 8% produce increasing effect

D – **T**

E – **F**   aphakes are responsive to parasympathomimetic agents

86.

A – **T**

B – **T**

C – **F**   neovascular glaucoma occasionally occurs after central retinal artery occlusion but not after branch retinal artery occlusion

D – **T**   posterior uveitis may lead to retinal ischaemia and thus to neovascular glaucoma

E – **T**   in carotico-cavernous fistula there is a reduced arterio-venous pressure gradient with resultant ocular ischaemia

87.

A – **T**

B – **T**

C – **F**   in POHS there is a chorio-retinitis

D – **F**   relapsing polychondritis is associated with scleritis

E – **T**

88.

A – **F**   it usually presents in teenagers and young adults

B – **F**   the eye is white

C – **F**   visual loss is most commonly due to macular oedema

D – **F**   it is usually bilateral

E – **F**   periocular steroids are particularly useful to avoid systemic
steroid therapy

89.

A – **F**   macular lesions are common

B – **F**   vitritis is common and may be severe

C – **F**   treatment does not eradicate the organism hence the
possibility of reactivation of infection

D – **F**   infection is occasionally acquired

E – **T**

90.

A – **F**   cytomegalovirus retinitis does respond to foscarnet as well as
to ganciclovir

B – **T**   cotton-wool spots may be due to vascular endothelial damage
by the HIV-1 virus or due to immune-complex deposition and
they do not indicate opportunistic retinal infection

C – **T**

D – **T**

E – **T**

91.

A – **F**   sympathetic ophthalmia may occur after any intraocular procedure although it is rare

B – **F**   Dahlen–Fuchs' nodules arise in the region of the retinal pigment epithelium

C – **T**

D – **F**   recurrent episodes of inflammation are common

E – **T**

92.

A – **F**   even with optimal therapy the visual prognosis is poor

B – **F**   ischaemic branch retinal vein occlusions are the characteristic finding

C – **T**

D – **T**

E – **T**

93.

A – **F**   Busacca nodules occur away from the iris margin

B – **F**   ocular involvement occurs in up to 30% of patients

C – **T**

D – **F**   the characteristic histopathological finding is non-caseating granulomas

E – **F**   hilar lymphadenopathy is usually asymptomatic

94.

A – **F**   cataract occurs in about 50% of cases

B – **F**   the keratitic precipitates are not affected by topical steroid therapy

C – **T**

D – **T**

E – **T**

95.

A – **F**   once vitreous haemorrhage occurs there must be proliferative retinopathy

B – **T**

C – **T**

D – **T**   although it is important to rule out a retinal tear

E – **T**   intraocular haemorrhage in association with subarachnoid haemorrhage is Terson's syndrome

96.

A – **T**

B – **F**   mid-peripheral ring scotomas are the earliest abnormalities of the visual field

C – **T**

D – **F**   nyctalopia (night blindness) is a very early feature

E – **T**

97.

A – **T**

B – **T**

C – **T**

D – **F**   the haemorrhagic retinopathy of occlusive carotid artery disease is due to poor central retinal artery perfusion and not central retinal vein occlusion

E – **T**

98.

A – **F**   it is most severe in the SC genotype

B – **T**

C – **F**   retinal neovascularization occurs on retinal vessels away from the optic disc

D – **T**

E – **T**   although retinal photocoagulation does reduce the frequency of vitreous haemorrhages

99.

A – **F**   proliferative retinopathy occurs in both
            non-insulin-dependent and insulin-dependent diabetes
B – **F**   up to 30% of patients with ischaemic maculopathy will
            develop proliferative retinopathy within 2 years and thus a
            major aspect of the management of patients with ischaemic
            maculopathy is the detection and treatment of proliferative
            retinopathy
C – **T**
D – **T**
E – **T**   patients from the Indian subcontinent have a high prevalence
            of diabetes and its complications

100.

A – **T**
B – **F**   the most commonly identified cause of branch retinal artery
            occlusion is emboli
C – **F**   central retinal artery occlusion not branch retinal artery
            occlusion occurs in giant cell arteritis
D – **F**   optic disc haemorrhages are not a feature of central retinal
            artery occlusion
E – **T**

101.

A – **T**
B – **T**   polycythaemia like other causes of hyperviscosity causes a
            slow flow retinopathy
C – **T**   anterior ischaemic neuropathy may complicate massive blood
            loss particularly if there is a pre-existing anaemia
D – **T**   vitamin B12 deficiency is associated with optic atrophy
E – **T**   sickle cell disease increases the risk of anterior segment
            ischaemia after squint surgery and after encirclement for
            retinal detachment repair

102.

A – T
B – T
C – T
D – F   Eales' disease is usually bilateral
E – F   retinal macroaneurysms commonly thrombose spontaneously

103.

A – T   men are 10 times more commonly affected than women
B – F   a 'smokestack' appearance is seen in the late venous phase of fluorescein angiography
C – F   spontaneous resolution occurs in about 90% of cases
D – F   choroidal neovascularization rarely complicates central serous retinopathy unless laser photocoagulation has been used
E – T

104.

A – T
B – F   Tay–Sachs disease causes a cherry-red spot at the macula
C – F   neurofibromatosis type 1 does not affect the retina
D – T
E – F   Laurence–Moon–Biedl syndrome causes a pigmentary retinopathy

105.

A – T
B – T   the Irvine–Gass syndrome is chronic cystoid macular oedema secondary to vitreous incarceration in a cataract section
C – T
D – T
E – F   cystoid macular oedema in association with diabetic retinopathy does not indicate macular ischaemia

106.
A – **T** in older patients retinal pigment epithelial detachments are frequently a sign of choroidal neovascularization
B – **T**
C – **T** particularly when associated with choroidal neovascularization
D – **F** they usually occur at the macula
E – **F** retinal pigment epithelial detachments indicate disease external to the retinal pigment epithelium which forms the outer blood–retinal barrier

107.
A – **T**
B – **T**
C – **F**
D – **F**
E – **F**

108.
A – **F** the pattern ERG assesses central retinal function
B – **F** the EOG is measured in the light and in the dark but not with flash stimuli
C – **F** the pattern VER cannot be obtained in the presence of opaque media but the flash VER will provide a measure of retinal function under such circumstances
D – **T**
E – **F** since the ERG is flat in retinitis pigmentosa the flash VER will also be abnormal

109.
A – **T**
B – **T**
C – **F** the Maddox rod test is a useful test of macular function in the presence of media opacity
D – **T**
E – **F** the Pulfrich phenomenon is a feature of unilateral optic nerve disease

110.

A – **F**   choroidal malignant melanoma is often associated with serous retinal detachment

B – **T**   spindle cells have a better prognosis than epithelioid cells

C – **T**

D – **T**

E – **T**

111.

A – **T**

B – **F**   in retrobulbar optic neuritis the optic disc is normal

C – **F**   in retrobulbar optic neuritis the optic disc does not leak fluorescein

D – **F**   a central scotoma is the usual field defect

E – **F**   there is usually an afferent pupillary defect

112.

A – **T**

B – **F**   if the ESR is raised it is likely to be arteritic anterior ischaemic optic neuropathy

C – **F**   visual loss usually develops abruptly

D – **F**   visual acuity usually does not change

E – **F**   on fluorescein angiography the optic disc shows a perfusion defect in the early phases and fluorescein leakage in the late phases

113.

A – **F**   colour vision is preserved in papilloedema until the late stages

B – **F**   spontaneous retinal venous pulsation is characteristically absent in papilloedema

C – **F**   the optic cup is well preserved until the disc swelling is marked

D – **F**   disc haemorrhages indicate acute vascular decompensation

E – **T**

114.

A – **F**   the esodeviation is the same for near and distance in congenital esotropia

B – **T**

C – **T**

D – **F**   in fully accommodative esotropia the deviation is fully controlled by refractive correction and surgery is not usually necessary

E – **T**

115.

A – **F**   the hyperdeviation in superior oblique palsy increases on gaze to the contralateral side

B – **T**

C – **F**   in sixth nerve palsy the esodeviation is greater for distance than for near

D – **T**

E – **T**

116.

A – **F**   only one active pupil is necessary to detect a relative afferent pupillary defect

B – **F**   optic nerve compression does not alter pupillary size

C – **T**   the Holmes–Adie pupil is hypersensitive to parasympathomimetic agents

D – **F**   cocaine is used to diagnose Horner's syndrome

E – **T**

117.

A – **F**   optic atrophy occurs late in chiasmal lesions

B – **T**   due to hemi-field slip

C – **F**   suprasellar masses infrequently cause raised intracranial pressure

D – **T**

E – **F**   bitemporal hemianopias may be confined to the central visual fields particularly in lesions compressing the posterior portion of the chiasm

118.

A – **T**

B – **F**   the temporal peripheral retina is predominantly involved

C – **F**   phenylephrine 2.5% should be used in babies to reduce the chances of systemic side-effects

D – **T**

E – **F**   stage 5 disease is the severe cicatricial stage and requires vitreo-retinal surgery if treatment is to be undertaken

119.

A – **T**   hence the need to initiate screening soon after birth

B – **F**   ocular albinism is either autosomal recessive or X-linked

C – **T**

D – **F**   the ERG is normal in delayed visual maturation

E – **T**

120.

A – **T**

B – **T**

C – **T**

D – **T**

E – **T**